Come
Home
to
Hope

Come Home to Hope

Sharon Hoffman

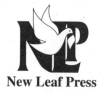

New Leaf Press

First printing: January 1999

ISBN: 0-89221-471-6
Library of Congress Number: 99-070072

Cover by Janell Robertson
Cover art by Kit Hevron Mahoney

Printed in the United States of America.

Acknowledgments

My heart holds dear all the precious ones in my life who have helped to make these pages a reality . . . many thanks from my heart go out:

To my husband, Rob, for giving me daily gifts of love, encouragement, and perspective. The greatest comfort in my life is having you by my side!

To Mindy, Missy, and Mike — how grateful I am to be your mom. You three bring chaos and comfort to my life . . . I love both!

To Dana Grimes for your polished writing contribution, and especially for your sustaining prayer, perseverance, and *pushing*. (You always seem to know when I need the latter!)

To my dear CCBC gals for carving out periods of quiet for me and for being an awesome "test group" for much of this material. Your lives verify God's comfort!

To the New Leaf Press family! You heard my passion and have been great each step of this project. I'm grateful to partner with such a godly, fun-loving team.

To Florence Littauer for your enthusiasm right from the start! You and Marita truly *wanted* me to write this series. You're the best!

To Marabel Morgan, whose teachings when I was just a newly-wed spawned much of my learning for loving my husband and my home.

And to you, dear reader friend, may God truly be the comfort of your heart and of your home.

Introduction

Welcome! Make yourself at home! If we were actually sitting across from each other in my cozy little parlor that I call the "welcoming room," I just know we'd become good friends. As you look around the room you would notice many gifts given to me by precious family and friends. It's with these cherished items that I love to decorate. My home might not pass an interior designer's inspection, but these daily reminders of joy sure do pass my test!

You'd see a china tea cup and saucer from my friend Diana on the sofa table. Delicately, it awakens memories of our encouraging walks and talks over the years. Underneath the table, on a lower shelf, lies a silk bouquet of long-stemmed peonies tied with iridescent organza. They were given to me as I stepped off the airplane by two effervescent ladies who met me at the airport in Richmond. Hard to believe such a delicate gift fared so well four flights later! But, I'm grateful they did — their beauty is now a constant reminder of new friends who were sensitive to my needs. Nearby, there's a little inspirational book with words of hope for me at a time when sweet Denise knew I really need affirmation.

It's not the gifts that matter most. It's the giving, caring, loving, endearing ways others have offered hope to me. The trust. The friendship. The interest shown. The timely encouragement . . . just b'cuz!

Yes, if you came to my home in person today, I'd tell you how glad I am you came! I'd throw a little "party of two" in your honor! Let's envision it. Candles would be lit! The flowers in the glass vase on the table would be for you! The pink cellophane-wrapped package by the door is for you to take with you as you leave. We'd chat endlessly about how similar we are and of our many common interests. I'd let you know how much I care about you just because you are YOU!

If you came over, it would be okay if you noticed the broken rocking chair and the throw rug that hides a stain here and there, I'd want you to know that nothing is too good for you — you are worth it! I'd hope you would feel how incredibly special you are! To me. To your friends and family. To God. He loves you and will never leave you. He offers you hope today. Hope that will help you hold on, even if you are at the end of your rope.

"But Christ as a son over his own house; whose house we are, if we hold fast the confidence and the rejoicing of the hope firm unto the end" (Heb. 3:6).

Your home, dear friend, is never without hope with God on your side. Read on to renew your hopes and dreams for your home. Until we have that parlor chat face to face, take hope in knowing you are loved. I love you; God loves you. Oh, how He loves you and me! Take comfort, you're about to see how I've learned from experience, you CAN "Come Home to Hope."

Come Home to Hope

Close Couples' Comfort Kit

"You love your husband very much, don't you?" I was asked one day after speaking at a workshop. Thinking about the day I stood in pure white at the altar as a bride, I answered an effervescent "YES!"

When Rob and I married 27 years ago, we committed to be faithful to each other and we have been. We promised to love one another with all our heart. And we have tried. Early on, we became aware that we both had much to learn about love — the real kind of love.

By the grace of God and armed with His strength, Rob and I have found that true love means giving ourselves to one another as Christ gave himself to us. That is, each putting the other's welfare and happiness above our own.

The Comfort Every Woman Craves

Psychologists tell us that a woman's most basic need is to feel secure love. This is the foremost comfort every woman craves in marriage. I've never met a woman who doesn't. Next to warm sexual love, a man needs admiration and approval. If your husband's coals of love have been dormant for a long time, it may take more than a spark to re-light his fire of love for you . . . especially if he's been burned before. But, it is possible.

How simple it would have been for Rob and I to go to a bookstore and come home with a manual containing master blueprints for our marriage. We would have followed the plan step by step. But there was no such book. That's no big surprise to anyone, now is it?

So, when our marriage had many more downs than ups during the eighth year, we had to admit we weren't doing well. On the course we were heading, there would not have been a "ten years from now." Something had to be done.

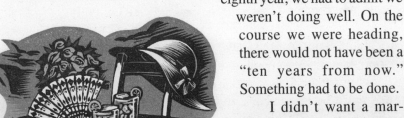

I didn't want a marginal marriage; I wanted the best. I made a conscious decision that something had to be done — and I knew it had to start with me.

I studied; I counseled; I became aware of the differences between the sexes. I read at night until I was cross-eyed. As I began to live by the principles I was learning, little things began changing. Almost immediately, Rob and I began to smile at each other. Our marriage was actually fun again. Romance returned. I almost felt like we were dating again.

One evening during a fun family time, we all four found ourselves laughing and frolicking on the floor. Catching his breath Rob said, "It's been a long, long time since we've heard a good laugh like that around here."

How sad, I thought with deep pangs of regret. But, I knew it was true. Rob was right, it had been way too long. I became more determined than ever to do something about it! As *I* changed, my husband's attitude toward me changed, too. I could hardly believe the communication and intimacy we began sharing.

My disposition became one of relaxed confidence. I had never enjoyed my marriage so much. Rob began to build shelves for me and do things spontaneously again. As I admired and appreciated his work he would think up more and more to do for me!

I am so grateful that I came out of that pit of self-pity and into a life that is such a joy and solidly stable. What I learned helped me to change (and continues to do so) from an independent, self-righteous mother and wife, into a new person. I realize now that I certainly had not lost my individuality or identity. I finally found it! Along with comfort and security!

Here it is over 25 years after I began applying the principles I've learned about true love. Just a few months ago, one night as I was drifting off to sleep, Rob nudged me. I asked him what was wrong or if there was something he needed. Pulling me close to him, my megaman husband whispered, "Just want you to know that I love you and I'm glad you love me." He rolled over and went right to sleep.

Now, maybe your husband wakes you up every night in the middle of a dream just to tell you he loves you, but mine sure doesn't. In the darkness I lay savoring that moment over and over for a long time afterward. Oh, the sweet comfort words of love bring!

Even if your marriage has no yellow warning lights flashing like mine did those first few years, the following "Close Couple's Comfort Kit" can guide you to redo, remake, repair, or remodel any marriage. Essentially, when you begin any home repair, you're on the careful lookout for what needs to be fixed. Do the same with your marriage. You locate the cracks and flaws and do what it takes to fix them. This kit will help you "get it together" or simply keep it together!

Use these tools as principles to rebuild your home. Every mistake has a positive quality in it. The changes in your marriage will be dramatic. You will be thrilled. Your husband will be thrilled! He will even be eager to apply the principles personally when he sees what is happening inside and outside of you. Your marriage can truly come alive . . . that's a promise.

The Close Couples' Cozy Comfort Kit

TOOL # 1 — RECOGNIZE THAT *YOU* ARE NOT PERFECT.

If you are a woman who truly desires that you and your husband can build a home of comfort, there are some issues in your *own* life that first must be hammered out. Recognize the attitudes and actions in yourself that need to be changed first.

Only when I was willing to admit my individual faults was my marriage relationship able to really change for the better. Trying to overcome selfishness in my own strength just made me want to give up. How hard it is for many of us "good wives" to admit that we are not perfect.

I had always been brought up to be good, kind, and religious. So much so, that it was very humbling to deal with the uncleansed areas of my life. The hard, cold truth was a little threatening,

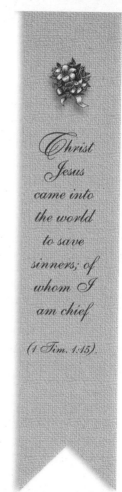

Christ Jesus came into the world to save sinners; of whom I am chief

(1 Tim. 1:15).

but my pride needed to be broken down.

This first stage takes time. Allow God to bring to your mind any unconfessed sin. Inner change came to me only as I was willing to commit my life to the Lord and ask for His help. I had to learn to agree with Paul when he said, "Christ Jesus came into the world to save sinners — of whom I am the worst" (1 Tim. 1:15), and James, "Humble yourselves before the Lord" (James 4:10). Believe me, it's much easier to humble *yourself* than it is to have God humble you.

In the early years of my marriage I used to think of myself as a loving wife and mother who didn't raise her voice and coped beautifully with difficult situations. Of course, this was not a true perception.

A more realistic observation came from my husband after days

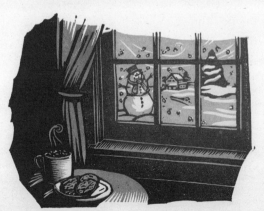

when a cloud of tension hung over our home. We went through the motions that everything was fine, but knew it wasn't. There was a barrier between us. The barrier was turning into thick walls.

As weeks turned into years, things got worse. Those walls in our home not only became uncomfortable, they were insurmountable. I wasn't sure what caused them and certainly did not know how to make them go away. But, I knew I didn't like them there. Helpless and unhappy, I felt up against an enemy I could not define or defy.

In a few short years I had allowed a negative, critical spirit to permeate my heart and become our home's atmosphere. Staring at the television I felt myself sitting and sighing day after day. I yearned for Rob to take me in his arms as the hero on the tube took the heroine in his.

I felt empty inside. I was afraid to be alone with my thoughts. I longed for something more. What was the answer? I began to search the Scriptures. I knew Jesus said He came to give us abundant life (John. 3:34) and that sounded so good to me. I didn't want to just live, I wanted to live abundantly.

This home repair "kit" is not intended to be the ultimate authority on marriage. Far from it. I don't pretend to have automatic, ready-to-wear answers for every marriage problem. I do believe with all my heart that it is possible for almost any wife to revive romance, break down communication walls, and return the sizzle to her marriage. And do so in just a few short weeks' time!

But you must first recognize your own arrogance and pride. Take a long look in your heart's full-length mirror. That's what I did to begin changing my life for the better. We can all profit so much from the beauty that humility brings.

The changes in your own life will bring about change in tangible ways in your husband. Instead of working on him, we must work on *ourselves* first. Backing your mate into a corner of your house would only bring reactions in anger, not actions of love.

Decide if you want to improve your marriage situation. Are you willing to do what God wants for your life, or are you going to continue to redo, redecorate, and remodel your partner? It is really up to you. You are to recognize *your* heart defects, not his!

Is it God's purpose that you have a positive, happy, exemplary marriage as a testimony of His goodness? It sure is! Don't put your faith in a pseudo cure-all or quick fix. Lasting change comes only from above, not from without . . . and it begins with your willingness to recognize that you can't do it by yourself.

TOOL #2 — REFRAIN FROM BLAME!

We women rationalize why we *need* to nag, blame, and find fault; after all, isn't all that in our job description? It's like we appoint ourselves to instruct, to remind, to guide . . . sounds more like to "control."

Maybe you are like me. I used to gather up all Rob's faults with the fervor of adding bricks to a stone wall. The walls I built became bitter barricades that only hindered effective communication and affection.

Tear down those walls today! Break down barriers by forgiving, apologizing, and most of all — loving. Because of past bad habits of seeing only negative, you may have to look long and hard to find the good in your mate. Hear me, if you don't . . . there are a lot of other women out there who will!

Even though I have taught these lessons and know them to be true, I still pick up bricks and build walls every now and then. I whine. I compare. I blame. I wail, "How come I'm the only one married to a man who isn't home at 6:00 for dinner every night? Why doesn't someone else at the office go in and check on emergencies that arise? Why does he say he's going to be gone only an hour and then stays gone half the day? How come every other wife has her expectations met?"

Sound familiar to anyone? Whew, with friends like that, what husband needs an enemy? You see how easy it is to find fault? Learn the lesson of "RE-FRAIN" before it is too late.

My friend who lives nearby tried to "help" her husband for years by criticizing, even often sarcastically saying, "If this situation or trait in you

Break down barriers by forgiving, apologizing, and most of all — loving.

doesn't improve, I just don't think I want to be married to you anymore."

She no longer has to worry. Sadly, they have been divorced a year now. On what would have been her wedding anniversary my friend lamented to me that her greatest regret was being upset and uptight about things that she realized later really didn't matter. She realized too late. But, you don't have to. Refrain from making repeated painful remarks that demean and that kill love.

Thank your Father in heaven for your mate and for the *positive* things you see in him. Philippians 4:8 directs our attention to a check-list of the good in others: "Finally, brothers, whatever is true, whatever is noble, whatever is right, whatever is pure, whatever is lovely, whatever is admirable — if anything is excellent or praiseworthy — think about such things."

No, it isn't easy. But, by an act of your will, you can *choose* to think on the positive in your man. When you read this passage over, can't you find the good things worthy of praise in your husband? Dwell on these things! The way to be happy in any relationship is to let go of the misunderstandings, arguments, or expectations. In five years, is it really going to matter anyway?

Not everything unpleasant that happens in life has to be someone's "fault." We spend our lives wanting people to act a certain way or fit a specific mold and when they're not — we blame, we fight, we hammer at them. I challenge you to go an entire week without any expectations from your spouse. Let go of them! When you free him to be as he is, then you, too, are freed! Free from the binding chains of expecting things to be like the Cinderella Syndrome. Holding on to unrealistic expectations is not true unconditional love.

Approach this exercise as you would any other. Getting started is the hardest. Remember: place no expectations on your husband. Any at all. Don't expect him to be on time. Don't expect him to be courteous. And guess what? Don't you be surprised when (not if) he is humble, gracious, and kind.

After a week, the exercise gets easier. Your frustration level will lower. Your marriage won't be problem-free, just a lot more fun. Instead of agitated toward each other, you'll both be a lot more accepting of each other. True happiness in marriage comes not when we get rid of all our problems, but when we let go of all our pre-conceived expectations. You will soon discover that marriage can be more of bliss . . . and less of a battle.

Marriage was never intended to be a reform school. If you married your man with the hope of "correcting all his problems," you've been courting

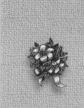

Marriage was never intended to be a reform school.

a possible disastrous future together. What did not change before marriage is not likely to change at all unless you give him the freedom to change. Maybe it's you who will change . . . you might realize he didn't need to so badly after all!

It's much more important to be kind than to be right!

TOOL #3 — REMEMBER BACK TO WHEN YOU FIRST FELL IN LOVE.

Remember what it was about your mate that you fell in love with in the first place? Begin by going back to that moment when you first saw that guy who is now your husband. Where was he? What was he dressed like? How did he act, talk, walk, comb his hair?

Remember? Oh, he was perfect. Not one flaw. You talked on the phone for hours. He held doors open for you. You wrote his name on every piece of paper you could find. You talked about this guy to everyone else constantly. He was your last thought at night and your first thought each morning. You were sure you were falling in love!

Remember what *you* looked and acted like when he first met you? Or how about when he'd pick you up for dates? Remember those long baths and how much time you took getting ready? You met him at the door with powder, perfume, and pizzazz!

Well, what did you look like last night when he came home? Scary thought, isn't it? It's no wonder the honeymoon is over! I'm not saying we gals have be groomed and gorgeous every evening to meet our husbands at the door a la gypsy outfits with beads, bangles, and bare skin.

However, as one man related to me recently, a man does want to come home to a *woman*. That's what he was attracted to when he noticed you in the first place. Femininity. Men are attracted to whatever is the opposite of a man. Femininity is the tender, gentle quality found in a woman's appearance, mannerisms, and nature. Femininity is *accenting* the differences between yourself and men, not the similarities.

You need not be beautiful to have the charm of femininity. I've known men who think their wives are absolutely beautiful even when a woman is so homely that the fact cannot be overlooked! He's finding her tenderness and loving ways *very* attractive to him. Loud, dominating, slap-you-on-the-back, obnoxious women are not feminine. To a man, they are screamers, unrefined, vulgar, and unattractive.

Analyze your feminine manner. Work on your weak points. Try it for at least a month. Watch how

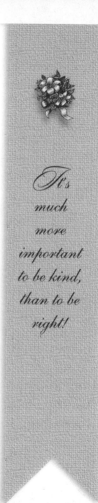

It's much more important to be kind, than to be right!

your husband adores you for trying! His natural impulse to provide and protect will be at an all-time high. Femininity sharply defines the difference between men and women, enhancing the attraction one for another.

In the excerpt from a letter that follows, notice how a young wife from Texas fights back sarcasm, aggressiveness, and humiliation:

"I came home from the retreat, and as I looked in the kitchen window, I saw TONS of boxes strewn all over my kitchen . . . the kitchen that I had just worked so hard to get clean the day before retreat. But I remembered your statement about the first four minutes being the most important, and I bit back the frustration and came in the house with a smile and a pleasant (if not totally sincere) hello.

Imagine my surprise when my husband took me by the hand and led me into the living room. Now, having just moved in recently, the living room was the catch all, with boxes almost to the ceiling (literally), and only a small path through them to the couch. So you can imagine how shocked I was when he led me in there, and all the boxes had been unpacked and things were put away, on the walls, etc. I was SO glad that I had kept my sarcastic greetings to myself! He had worked hard all day long trying to have the room finished before I came in, and all that was left was the empty boxes in my kitchen, which he promptly broke down and took out. We were able to have company that night without me being totally embarrassed about the state of my house, thanks to my wonderful husband!"

Thank you, Gina, for sharing with me and letting me use your learned lessons to help others. Gina's response in those first four minutes upon arriving home set the tone for the rest of the evening. She took the retreat advice seriously and it paid off immediately! A heated argument those first four minutes could have put a damper on the whole evening. So it is in the morning when your family gathers to touch base for the busy day. Send your husband off with feminine reminders of peace and harmony.

Remember those endearing qualities about your courtship — the way you were can become the way you *are!*

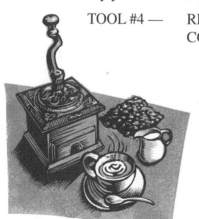

TOOL #4 — RE-OPEN THE LINES OF COMMUNICATION.

Re-open the lines of communication in your home. A woman expresses her love by words and expects words in return. That's not the way she always gets it. A man more often expresses his love by actions — bringing home the paycheck, sex, buying his wife a house or pots and pans. She wants words and tenderness; he gives her material goods. Is it any wonder that men and women have trouble communicating?

Is your marriage line of communication clogged from under use? It may be shut down to only a few drips a day. You can become a communication plumber and re-open backed-up draining by becoming a good listener. Anyone can talk, but true love really *listens*.

"Guess what, honey?" Jim exclaimed as he bounded in for dinner. "I finally landed the Morris account! What a stress that has been these past two months, but what a relief now."

In the midst of dinner preparation Lynn hastily asked, "Did you remember to pick up the dry cleaning on the way home?" She hadn't heard a word Jim said. He longed for her to be proud of his accomplishment. He was seeking perhaps the one thing that a man needs most from his wife — recognition and respect.

He didn't get it.

Being a sanguine in personality, as well as a speaker by profession, I understand Lynn's predicament. For years I would preoccupy myself when Rob talked or interrupt with a story of my own. I found out, by trial and error, that Rob wants my whole attention. Not half. Not correct or condemn. He wants me to look at him, concentrate on him, hang on every word.

He needs me to be his number one fan and prove it to him by being a good listener. One evening not so long ago before he was to speak at his alma mater, Rob asked me to listen to the message he'd worked so hard on. So I listened. Not just once, but three times I listened to it.

As Rob went through each point, example, quote, I did not sew or look at magazines or file my fingernails. I gave him my undivided attention for almost an hour with my eyes transfixed directly on his. When it came time to present it to the college student body the next morning, I could tell he felt confident. I was thankful I had listened intently. He needed my attention to add affirmation.

Remember something Gary Smalley said in *Love Languages,* "Non-verbal communication is the most powerful part of any message we communicate. Tone of voice, eye contact, facial expressions, show of interest, sincere desire, and patience with the answers."[1]

To me that says that communication is actually listening to the other person's needs as well as what they are verbally saying. It has a lot of everyday practical faces and sounds. I have heard a man say, "Why talk to my wife? She won't even quit doing dishes," or "She's always on the phone when

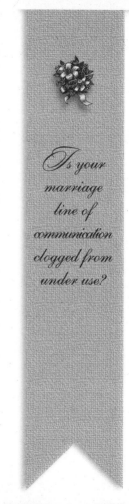

Is your marriage line of communication clogged from under use?

I come home." Message: "I'm insignificant."

I often hear women say, "He just keeps on reading the paper when I tell him about my day," or "I can't unglue him from the TV." Message: "I'm uncherished." Listening, eyeball to eyeball, gives the feeling that "I am on your team and I will help you get where you're going."

The love communicated in greetings and partings is especially important. If you did not experience strong communication bonding in your family of origin, you can start by pausing to take time to greet those whom you have been separated from, let them know that they are important and you are glad to see them again.

Partings are as important as greetings. Make the time to walk your husband to the door as he leaves. Let him know you eagerly await his return. Then stand on the porch waving. (The first time you do this, he may drive back into the driveway thinking you are motioning that he forgot something — my Rob did!) He will leave feeling affirmed and cherished from this enthusiastic parting. He hopes to return home to such a warm and welcoming wife! Work and schedules are accelerated to the extent that this may not be feasible every single day, but in some way we need to take the time to greet those from whom we've been separated.

I know I am not the most beautiful woman that ever walked the face of this earth . . . or the most talented . . . or the most wonderful, but I sure feel as though I am in Rob's eyes when we are reunited at the end of the day. We communicate. Especially in airports. We communicate! You should see us after a couple days' separation. Deportment goes straight out the window! We cannot restrain the huge smiles across our faces when our eyes meet down that long corridor. I usually jump up and down, expressing sheer glee just to be back together. That's communication!

The "macho" man image is really a myth carried over from the fifties. Contrary to popular opinion, a man doesn't enjoy a knock-down, drag-out fight with his wife. Whether its tears or shouting, he simply does not know how to cope with such emotion. To protect his self-esteem, he fights back.

When I'm mad at Rob, I warn him ahead of time. I say something like, "I'm getting too emotional and growly. I need some time out!" Sometimes I go out on the porch alone, or downstairs to cry and feel sorry for myself. After I calm down and regain my composure, I return to carry on the conversation.

I find that it is best to then say what I have to say; then forgive and forget. Communication is not to sulk, nag, or refuse sex as a punishment. Playing the silent martyr takes too much tremendous emotional effort for me. It only intensifies the problems and turns molehills into mountains anyway. That type of silence is not really golden.

When you communicate by sharing, not shoving, you'll see how easy it will be for your husband to reciprocate. When I built that "wall" of Rob's faults, they became bitter barricades that only hindered effective communication and affection.

Those walls had to come down. By apologizing, forgiving, and — most of all — tenderness, down they came.

If you are like me with past bad habits of seeing only the negative, you may have to work long and hard at finding the good in your husband. If you don't, hear me again . . . there are plenty of other women out there who will!

Oh sure, you will have many opportunities to "correct" your husband. Occasionally I slip back into my old faultfinding ways. When I do, the atmosphere in our home goes *kerplunk*. Everyone ends up being miserable — including me. If I want to spend my time looking at Rob's bad side, I'm sure I can find it. When I spend time criticizing him in my heart, naturally it comes across in my attitude.

A woman with a tender, loving heart knows that it is impossible to feel better about herself at the expense of her husband. We've all been uncomfortable around women who have to be "right" all the time.

They jump in to correct their husband's story just to prove they know how "it really was."

Just last night I noticed the expression on a man's face as his wife "jumped in there." He stopped talking and let her finish. After all, she obviously was out to prove she was smarter, wiser, and a much better storyteller. The rest of the evening was very uncomfortable. This belittled husband said very little and was clearly embarrassed.

When my conversation focuses on Rob's good, he never tires of hearing it. Neither do I. My critical communication can crush his spirit quicker than anything. It's amazing to me, however, how my positive conversation *to* Rob encourages positive communication *from* Rob. I am keeping a list in my heart of treasures he has said to me in recent months, such as "I love you more and more all the time" and "I sure have enjoyed living with you these 27 years" and "There's honestly no one in this world I'd rather be with than you."

These loving endearments echo in my ears. Just as Rob never tires of hearing how loved he is, neither do I. *That's communication!*

When you communicate by sharing, not shoving, you'll see how easy it will be for your husband to reciprocate.

TOOL #5 — RENEW AND REVIVE ROMANCE

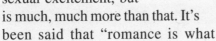

Romance, you say, in *my marriage?* What *is* romance, anyway? If we are honest, it has an element of sexual excitement, but is much, much more than that. It's been said that "romance is what makes two married people sit in the middle of a bench when there's plenty of room at both ends."

What, then, do you do when the romance has gone out of your marriage? Answer: You go right back to the One who created marriage and the beauty of sex. To God. It was His idea in the first place. It is to be guilt-free and wholesome. Sex is God's lovely wedding gift to every bride and groom. What a great romantic!

Sex is not everything in marriage, so I am not trying to exaggerate its importance. But, it is an integral part of the marriage relationship when there is a mating of spirit with spirit. We don't need to be ashamed to talk about what God was not ashamed to create. God conceived the idea by creating the two sexes instead of just one.

Imagine the fun and games Adam and Eve had in the garden. There were no marriage manuals or counselors to consult. Imagine Adam exclaiming, "Where have you been all my life!" (That's a rather loose translation; it was actually, "Bone of my bones, flesh of my flesh.")

God provided someone to meet Adam's needs. There they were — naked, beautiful, perfect, trusting one another. They fit together perfectly! When a relationship is built on standards of trust, commitment, understanding, and unselfish devotion, romance flourishes. If your intimate love life is not all you want it to be, you can do something about it today. It is surprising how uneducated many husbands and wives are concerning sex. In many cases a re-educating about the basics is all that is needed to relieve tension in the romance department.

There are so many good Christian manuals that deal specifically with the physical mechanics of sex that both you and your husband might find helpful. Attitudes that may have affected your sex life for years can be altered with proper wholesome sex education.

TOOL #6 — RELINQUISH YOUR HUSBAND TO HIS RIGHTFUL OWNER.

Your husband will never truly be yours until you have first given him to God. You do not *own* him! He is yours only when you are willing to let him go wherever God calls him and to do whatever God wants him to do!

When I got married I had some preconceived notions of what the future would be. You might say I was bitten by a bug with Cinderella symptoms. This "disorder" leaves one with delusions that hinder the thinking processes. In my case, my thinking was stymied, all right. I dreamed only of living in a white, two-story house on an acre of ground, with tall, rustling trees in the backyard, and flower gardens surrounding the entire setting. There would be soft, fluffy snow in the winter and green fields filled with clover in the summer. Everyone would arrive at our home for the holidays. We'd have a full, long table with turkey and the trimmings.

When I discarded this unrealistic dream I was a happier, better wife. I found that through the years this dream got in my way and made me less adaptable than I should have been. To be adaptable, *make your dreams portable.* Plan to be happy anywhere — on a mountain or in a burning desert; in poverty's vale or abounding in wealth. Why is this so important? Because your husband is not yours.

Don't be rigid and set in your ways. Determine to adjust to life's circumstances. God's ways are not always our ways. A contented spirit during times that require flexibility is a rare quality in a woman. It is, however, a quality that is treasured by men. To be adaptable you have to be unselfish, care more about others than yourself, and put your marriage in top priority. Yes, I discarded my unrealistic dreams but held on to the dreams that I felt were non-negotiable. And you know what? Many, many of them have come true! *When you cast your bread upon the waters, it comes back to you buttered!* Don't lose sight of what is honestly a God-given goal or dream. But, relinquish people to the One who can make those dreams come true.

Just as Abraham had to open his hands and yield on that ancient altar the one thing that kept him from complete surrender, so we have to yield. Your husband is your husband. Not your possession. His first love is God. Not you. Don't make him choose between you two. The greater the possessiveness, the greater the pain in letting go.

Often we are hindered from giving up our treasures out of fear for their safety or security. But, wait a minute! Isn't everything safe and secure in the hands of God? In fact, nothing or no one is really safe or secure *unless* they are totally committed to God. No child. No dream. No job. No romance. No friend. No house. Especially, no husband.

What does God want us wives to do? I've had

To be adaptable, make your dreams portable. Plan to be happy anywhere.

to do it a zillion times. Let go. Release the grip. Turn loose. No matter how you phrase it, it still creates panic and fear in our hearts. "But, my husband is not a godly man and I cannot trust him," you say. God can do a much better work in his life if you step out of the way.

Wise was the older woman years ago who gave me some very good advice when she said, "Sharon, it is your job to make Rob happy; not holy!" It's one of those great paradox lessons. The more I let go of Rob, the more he truly becomes "mine." Mine in love, mine in laughter, mine in life! Like one of those "less is more" admonitions. I've tried clinging . . . Rob just struggles hard to get away. When I release, he seeks me out all the more.

We're told that "whosoever shall *lose* his life shall *find* it." I've had to learn that lesson the hard way, but have found it to be absolutely true. Can losing actually produce gain? It sure can! How unpopular that philosophy is today. Somehow people can't handle losing. We just are not taught that losing could be a positive thing.

From our rat-race perspective, it seems that Jesus must have had a few things mixed up. To us, losing is unpleasant. Losing means failure. To us maybe; not to Christ. Many women frantically scurry around looking everywhere for ways to improve intimacy with their husband, when the secret has been right there all along. The secret is in the yielding.

One woman wrote me from Ohio that she and her husband were

seriously thinking of separation. They were both miserable. One evening she stopped the packing and started praying. "O God, help me to lose my husband (to You) so I can find him!" What a freedom she discovered in letting go! I love how she concludes her letter, "I took my hands off of my husband, now *he can't keep his hands off me!"*

Of course there was much more to her letter as this young woman told their story, but let me just include the poem entitled "Treasures" — it says it all.

Treasures

One by one He took them from me. All the things I valued most
Until I was empty-handed; Every glittering toy was lost.

And I walked earth's highways, grieving, In my rags of poverty.
Till I heard His voice inviting "Lift your *empty* hands to Me!"
          (italics mine)

So I held my hands toward heaven, And He filled them with a store
Of His own transcendent riches Till my hands could hold no more.

And at last I comprehended With my stupid mind and dull
That God could not pour His riches Into hands already full.
        by Martha Snell Nicholson[2]

TOOL #7 — RESTORE RESPECT.

What is a man proud of? A man needs to feel proud of his masculine role by meeting these five masculine needs:

1. A man needs to be admired.
2. A man needs to know he is appreciated.
3. A man needs companionship.
4. A man needs to be prayed for.
5. A man needs to be affirmed for who he is.

Respect is restored in a marriage when a wife fills her husband's emotional cup with admiration. He needs to hear that you *really need him*. So deep is his need to feel needed as a man and to serve as a man, that when he is no longer needed he may question his reason for living. This affects a man's tender feelings for his wife since his romantic feelings partly arise from her need to be protected, sheltered, and cared for.

Unfortunately, we women too often meet so many of our own needs ourselves that our husbands fail to receive the honor they crave. They long to meet our needs and serve as the protector, sheltering you from harm, danger, or difficulty. Respect is shown to a man by a strong, wise woman who has learned to trust her husband.

Many men will do just about anything to gain the admiration of others, especially their families. They will search and search for some-one to love and respect them. *Make sure that someone is you.* Honor his position as the head of the family and teach your children to do so. If you do feel that he is about to make a mess of things, first hear his point of view. Don't hasten to jump in. Spend a lot of time thinking before you step in and advise; then outline a course for him to follow. Not man to man. But, as a woman who loves, respects, and cares.

Let go of the reigns in the family. Turning over rightful control to your husband is extremely important as a basis for couples to achieve a genuinely satisfying relationship in marriage. Follow your husband when he leads. Remember: if we wives would be better followers, many husbands would become better leaders.

Don't expect every decision your husband makes to make sense to you. Sometimes decisions may defy logic. If he is leaning on the

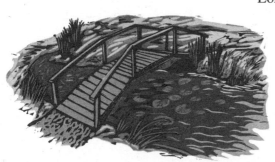

Lord concerning a decision and not just trying to be the "big kahuna," ask your Heavenly Father to guide him. If his plans do not make sense to you, nor his judgment appear the least bit sound, perhaps it isn't.

But, the ways of God don't always follow logic. God may lead your husband into problems or allow him to even fail for a wise reason. Let God try him in the refiner's fire if He so chooses. And get out of the way! If you don't, *you* will end up getting burnt!

When I step aside and let God do what He so chooses in the lives of those I love, things often turn out right in a surprising way. When Rob senses that I trust his overall judgment and motives, it makes him feel so responsible that he makes sure he does the right thing. Turning things over to him through the years has built my confidence in him and his confidence in himself.

Have faith in the principle that God has placed your husband at the head and commanded you to obey him, as stated in the Bible in Ephesians 5 and 1 Peter 3. The home can only fulfill its true purpose when it is God-controlled. Leave Jesus Christ out of your home and it loses its meaning. But follow Christ's plan for the home, and He will make it the greatest haven this side of heaven. If you can't trust your husband concerning an issue, you can always trust God!

As a wife, doing recreational things with your husband can be a real key to companionship. This doesn't mean you have to take up hunting or basketball, but picking an interest of his can pay rich dividends: walking, swimming, golf, antique hunting, fishing, gardening, refinishing furniture together — just to name a few.

By taking advantage of a variety of ways to participate in activity

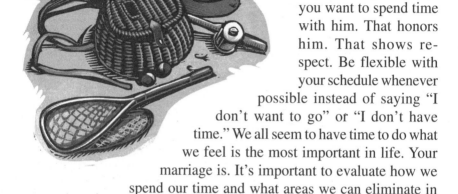

with your husband, you are showing him that you want to spend time with him. That honors him. That shows respect. Be flexible with your schedule whenever possible instead of saying "I don't want to go" or "I don't have time." We all seem to have time to do what we feel is the most important in life. Your marriage is. It's important to evaluate how we spend our time and what areas we can eliminate in order to schedule quality time with our mate.

Many Christians have mastered the art of looking spiritual and happy on the outside. But once they enter their homes, they take off the masks and let down their guards. They take out their frustrations on the people who mean the most to them. For many, that frustration is taken out on their spouse so that the children are "spared."

Respect gives your husband permission to be himself. You, as the wife, become the "safe" person to whom he can express himself and know he will be understood, trusted, and not condemned for it. The secret of empowering a man with respect is not trying to change him or improve him. When a man feels loved, trusted, respected, and appreciated — automatically he begins to change, to grow, and to improve in the very areas you desire him to.

Many times I have mistakenly tried to "fix" Rob and he responded by defending himself. The behavior I was trying to fix stayed the same. He did not feel accepted so he actively or passively resisted. He only felt controlled and corrected.

The best way to help a man grow is to let go of trying to change him, and pray, pray, pray. In prayer, I accept Rob's feelings, actions, or "imperfections." Praying to God out loud, if possible, gives me a greater awareness of the truth that God is in control, not me. Rather than disrespect, Rob appreciates my vulnerability and sensitivity when he knows I have taken a matter to the Lord. Remember: Men are more willing to say "yes" if they are respected and know they have the freedom to say "no."

TOOL # 8 — REFUSE TO CHOOSE DIVORCE AS AN OPTION.

The best place to make this choice is before the church bells begin to ring and you're walking down the aisle. Unfortunately, not every couple does. When couples fall in love we feel as though we will be happy forever. We cannot imagine not loving our partner or ever being with someone else. It is a magical time when everything in the relationship is in harmony and works effortlessly.

Then we realize our partner is not as perfect as we thought. We have to work at love, getting along, and daily life. He isn't the man we thought we knew. In fact, he is from another planet! We discover our husband is flawed and makes mistakes. It is no longer easy to give love. Not only is it difficult . . . we do not always feel like giving love.

Love is seasonal. Summertime brings disappointments that must be up-rooted under the hot, sweltering heat of discouragement. Autumn's harvest is golden-rich and fulfilling. A more mature love grows and understands an abundance of hope and possibilities. There are the cold, difficult, barren winters. The weather changes again, and springtime comes. It is a time of relationship renewal and enjoyment of the union that love has created.

I have witnessed countless couples who have worked hard through all these seasons, year in and year out. *Commitment* is the common trait that I've observed that infused their marriages through difficulties in each season. Commitment. Strange, isn't it, that it all boils down to one word. Yet that one word is in short supply in many marriages.

We have to work at love, getting along, and daily life.

We are a culture that is used to getting what we want instantly. We hate waiting patiently — on anything. We can push a button to instantly raise our garage door, open our car, lock our house, cook an entire meal in just a few seconds. We don't want to wait. That takes commitment. There's that word again.

Are you committed? When you go through a difficult season in your marriage, your mate needs to hear words of commitment — not rejection. Each time you argue about a problem or disagree, do you threaten to leave? What a cruel tactic! It instills fear in your husband and erodes the security of your marriage.

Tell your husband how much you love him. Often. Many, many times. Not just in the peaceful seasons, but in the turbulent times. Assure your husband that you will remain loyal and true to the marriage covenant that you agreed to preserve when you said "I do." Never threaten to leave. (The exception here would be if you or your children are in danger of being harmed. Then go to a safe place and get help. Don't become a casualty or statistic. In the case of physical or psychological abuse, homosexuality, drunkenness, drugs, etc., separation may be necessary while searching for a redemptive solution.)

Make sure your husband knows that you are committed to your marriage, especially if you have threatened to leave him in the past. A wedding anniversary would be the opportune time to sweetly and sincerely demonstrate your devotion. Tell your husband that you would marry him all over again! Tell him that the idea of divorce is not even an option to you.

I listened to a dear young husband recently who, through tears, shared with me how his wife had come home and done just that. Weeping in humility and grace he took her in his arms and held her with a tenderness never before. This man's fears of losing his precious little wife were finally put to rest. To put it in his words, "I felt like a plant that had been placed out in the sun after being inside for a long, dark winter."

Don't believe the lies of Satan and society that say you can just marry someone else later if your marriage doesn't work out. Our culture wants you to believe that you can come out unscathed. I wish you could see the tears and heartache that Rob and I have witnessed during marriage breakups. God shuns divorce. He says so in Malachi 2:15-16. It was never His choosing from the very beginning.

Poor marriages are *caused* by not repairing the home — good marriages are *created* by building with these tools. Yes, you and your husband are in this thing together. If your roof springs a leak, you're

You both win or you both lose.

both going to get wet. And if enough water from the storms of life gets in, you're both going to drown. Either you both win or you both lose. There is no other option. Marriage demands the integrated efforts of both you and your husband.

The very best athletic teams understand that success is built on the strengths of all their players. The burly strongman may make fantastic tackles, but the small, agile player can sneak through the line without getting crunched. Games are won because they have developed a team approach where each player uses their God-given strengths.

So it is that marriage partners know where their strengths lie, as well as their corresponding weaknesses. They compensate for one another; they work together. It's two sides of the same coin. Through any dark season, refusal to even consider divorce as an option helps heal many wounds.

One last thought with this tool is something that I heard years ago. It went something like this: "The best thing you can do for your children is to love their father." The trust that you give your husband and your children when you make your commitment known will give your family some precious gifts. Gifts every family longs for: of feeling safe, secure, and strong.

Luke 1:37 tells us, *"For nothing is impossible with God."* You don't have a problem that He cannot work out — if you turn that problem over to God. It doesn't matter how painful your situation is, God cares. Tell Him about it (1 Pet. 5:6-7). Ask Him what to do (James 1:5-8). Be sure that what you think you hear Him say agrees with His written Word (John 8:31-32). Obey Him (John 7:17). Trust Him (Isa. 26:3-4). God won't always do *your* will. But when He doesn't, it is because He will do "immeasurably more than all we ask or imagine" (Eph. 3:20).

Henry Ford was asked on the occasion of his fiftieth wedding anniversary, "What is the formula for a good marriage?" He replied, "The same as for a successful car: stick to one model." That's great advice, Mr. Ford!

This World Is Not My Home

If I decided to build a house, what would my house look like? On paper, some kind of monstrosity, I'm sure! I would definitely need an architect who could draw not only an overall plan, but an extremely detailed one.

In a small town not too many miles from where I live, a superb home has just been completed. Master builders from all across the Midwest worked one

The best thing you can do for your children is to love their father.

entire year to finish this widely acclaimed home in time for the world's only living septuplets' first birthday. In fact, today is moving-in day for the now-famous McCaughey family. Completion of their home, which is three times the size of an average home, has been quite a feat — even for the most accomplished designers.

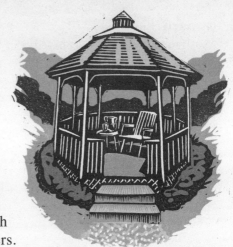

To build such a mammoth house required master builders. They had to plan in a most grandiose scale for a home that would meet the needs of seven toddlers who would someday become seven teenagers. Planning right along with the input of the parents, the contractor had to be one very patient builder. They longed for their house to be a place where the children could run, play, and grow up in private. "To be their home, not a museum," pleaded Kenny McCaughey.

I'm sure there are not many human architects anywhere willing to take on a solemn project like that. But that describes the Lord Jesus perfectly. Given complete control, He will build within us each a lovely house indeed! A house will stand the storms of life when Christ is not only our architect and builder, but the foundation as well.

Jesus does not want to just *lay* a foundation, but will *become* the foundation. "For no one can lay any foundation other than the one already laid, which is Jesus Christ" (1 Cor. 3:11). He desires to become the sure, secure foundation in the "ways" of your life.

So far in this book we've taken your old house, the "real you," and we've done a lot of remodeling and renovating. We've painted, planted some new shrubs, and repaired a few loose shutters on the outside. Inside, we've cleaned closets, dusted throughout, vacuumed under the sofa, and decorated with lovely touches to enhance the comfort level.

What we need now is the power. Without a power source for warmth, light, and air flow, your shell is nothing more than a glorified outhouse. Years ago I "plugged in" to the world's greatest power source. You can, too. Making the connection means abundant life for you. I'd love to show you how.

Opening the Door of Your Heart

Have you ever stood outside a friend's house knocking and ringing the doorbell until finally you left, assuming no one was at home? Jesus stands at the door of your heart today, dear friend (Rev. 3:20). He longs to dwell there through faith (Eph. 3:16-17). He longs to settle down and be at home. Christ will live in any human heart that welcomes him in through believing on Him.

It's your choice. The door of your heart represents that power of choice. No matter what sin or what pain there might be in your past, Jesus is ready to forgive and to make you whole (1 John 1:9). The love of Christ is clear in many passages in the Bible, perhaps the dearest in John 3:16: "For God so loved the world that he gave his one and only Son, that whoever believes in him shall not perish but have eternal life."

Oh, God's love for me! I never get over it. I hope I never do. Jesus said he came to give us an awesome, abundant life (John 10:10). But how do you plug into the power of the God of the universe? Thousands of years ago, Isaiah said, "Your iniquities have separated you from your God" (Isa. 59:2). Our sins, yours and mine, keep us away from God and his power. Oh, you may not feel like the "bad" in your life is too bad. I didn't either until I came across the truth in the Bible that astounds me.

They weren't gross sins, but I was guilty of them nonetheless. Worry, pride, gossip, and unbelief, to name a few. That was me . . . separated from God due to the fact that the penalty for sin is spiritual death according to Romans 6:23. But, there's good news, too, right in the same verse: "But the gift of God is eternal life in Christ Jesus our Lord."

Since I knew I could not personally bridge the wide gap to God by myself, that *is* good news. Great news! What's more, the Bible tells us how to accept that gift of eternal life. The verses in Ephesians 2:8 and 9 read, "For it is by grace you have been saved, through faith — and this not from yourselves, it is the gift of God — not by works, so that no one can boast."

Jesus spent a lifetime on this earth unselfishly healing broken lives and broken hearts. He then died so that we might live. He stands knocking at a symbolic door of our heart: "Here I am! I stand at the door and knock. If anyone hears my voice and opens the door, I will come in and eat with him, and he with me" (Rev. 3:20).

By faith, I opened my heart's door to Jesus when I was just a young child. For nearly 40 years, His free gift has been the source of my peace and joy. I am His very own child, spiritually born into the family of heaven with the promise of a heavenly home. Forever secure because of what Christ has done for me, there is not a chance of losing my eternal life because it has been paid for and secured

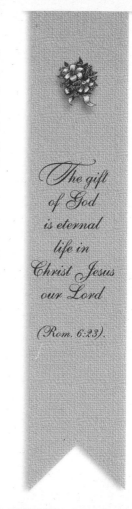

The gift of God is eternal life in Christ Jesus our Lord

(Rom. 6:23).

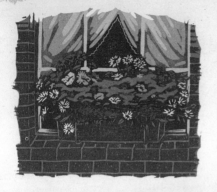

by what Christ did on the cross.

When a friend comes to your home with a special delivery, you can hardly wait to let him in. Now Jesus is asking to come into your heart as Lord and Savior. He stands knocking with a gift of incomparable value — that gift of eternal life! Won't you let Him come into your heart and life right now? If you believe that He died as the Savior for the sins of the world, invite Him in today.

Your Heart Becomes a Home

There are two kinds of re-decorating. Don't be satisfied with a new outer paint job and some temporary re-doing. Re-model from the ground (heart) up! Receive, accept the One, the only One, who can bring true comfort and give you life. Pascal once said, "There is a God-shaped vacuum in the heart of every man, which cannot be satisfied by any created thing, but only by God, the Creator." God is waiting and wanting to fill the vacuum of your heart.

Right now your heart can become a heart of confidence, calm, and comfort . . . instead of chaos. Jesus Christ promises these wonderful benefits to all who open their heart's door to Him.

Invite Him into your life. Simply open the door. The following is a suggested prayer that many women in my classes have used:

> "Dear Jesus, I need you. Thank You for loving me so much that You died on Calvary's cross. Right now, I open the door of my heart to invite you into my life as my personal Savior. I ask You to forgive my sins and make me the kind of person You want me to be. I love You, Lord, and I thank You. Amen.

I give you my word, dear reader, when you give your heart and life to Christ, there is no greater comfort to be found! Christ IS the great comforter. He alone will give the peace that I, too, had searched for all too long. He promises to settle in and be at home as the Lord of your heart. It's as though you transfer the title and deed over to Jesus Christ. Sign it over.

You will never be the same. You will never be sorry.

Transfer of the Title

As owner and master of my heart, Christ has the freedom to manage and operate my life as He chooses. It is no longer my responsibility to keep my heart what it ought to be. I couldn't live a pleasing Christian life in my own strength. It would be impossible.

The only way it really works is to give Christ full ownership — for time and eternity. God's Word assures me that He holds the deed to my heart firmly in His hands. Giving Him daily control makes sure that I do not take it back! He can do a much better job of taking care of my assets and liabilities than I ever could anyway.

The gift of salvation is not the last gift God offers us. It's the first. And it sets the pattern for all that follow. Salvation from sin's guilt is only the beginning. Take a look at all the other gifts He has freely bestowed upon us as His children:

First of all, I have *confidence* — the inner confidence that comes from God Himself. God has given us all we need to be confident. "God did not give us a spirit of timidity, but a spirit of power, of love and of self-discipline" (2 Tim. 1:7).

> *I am confident* that I am never alone because God has said, "Never will I leave you; never will I forsake you" (Heb. 13:5).

> *I am confident* that He will always provide for me. "I was young and now I am old, yet I have never seen the righteous forsaken or their children begging bread" (Ps. 37:25).

> *I am confident* that I can make it through whatever life brings my way for "I can do everything through him who gives me strength" (Phil. 4:13).

I am confident in my relationship with Christ, "I know whom I have believed, and am convinced that he is able to guard what I have entrusted to him for that day" (2 Tim. 1:12).

I am confident that I can trust God implicitly to be at work in my life. "My grace is sufficient for you, for my power is made perfect in weakness" (2 Cor. 12:9).

I am confident that I can rely on God, no matter what. "In quietness and trust is your strength" (Isa. 30:15).

Secondly, I have a *calm* that I can live in safety and without fear. "Do not fear, for I am with you; do not be dismayed, for I am your God, I will strengthen you and help you; I will uphold you with my righteous right hand" (Isa. 41:10).

I have a calm during the storms of life for God has promised, "When you pass through the waters, I will be with

I can do everything through him who gives me strength

(Phil. 4:13).

you; and when you pass through the rivers, they will not sweep over you" (Isa. 43:2).

I calmly do not have to be afraid when others attack me. "The Lord is a refuge for the oppressed, a stronghold in times of trouble" (Ps. 9:9).

I can know a calm and quiet in this noisy world. "Whoever listens to me will live in safety and be at ease, without fear of harm" (Prov. 1:33).

I can calmly face the future. " 'For I know the plans I have for you,' declares the Lord, 'plans to prosper you and not to harm you, plans to give you hope and a future' " (Jer. 29:11).

I can feel calm when I feel like I'm going to lose my mind! "And the peace of God, which transcends all understanding, will guard your hearts and your minds in Christ Jesus" (Phil. 4:7).

I have an unexplainable calm that nothing in this world can offer, for Jesus said, "Peace I leave with you; my peace I give you. I do not give to you as the world gives. Do not let your hearts be troubled and do not be afraid" (John 14:27).

Thirdly, I have unlimited *comfort* available to me. To belong to the Creator of the world, what could be a greater comfort? He knows me, sees me, cares for me, and loves me! (Ps. 147).

I have comfort because the comforter actually lives within my heart. "And I will ask the Father, and he will give you another Counselor to be with you forever — the Spirit of truth. The world cannot accept him, because it neither sees him nor knows him, But you know him, for he lives with you and will be in you" (John 14:16-17).

What comfort to know that God is in control. He's omnipotent, having all power (Luke 1:35); omnipresent, everywhere present at the same time (Psalm 139:7); and omniscient, all knowing (1 Cor. 2:10-11).

Comfort is mine when I am brokenhearted. "The sacrifices of God are a broken spirit; a broken and contrite heart, O God, you will not despise" (Ps. 51:17).

My heart is comforted when I realize that I am going to be with Jesus in

Do not let your hearts be troubled and do not be afraid

(John 14:27).

my heavenly home eternally. "We are confident, I say, and would prefer to be away from the body and at home with the Lord" (2 Cor. 5:8).

I am comforted in any circumstance when I feel like everything or everyone is against me. "If God is for us, who can be against us?" (Rom. 8:31).

I can think of nothing more comforting than realizing God is with me always. "Never will I leave you; never will I forsake you" (Heb. 13:5).

I find comfort in knowing that God's plan is not for me to fail, but to succeed. " 'For I know the plans I have for you,' declares the Lord, 'plans to prosper you and not to harm you, plans to give you hope and a future' " (Jer. 29:11).

Comfort is available during excruciatingly painful and trying times in my life. "And we know that in all things God works for the good of those who love him, who have been called according to his purpose" (Rom. 8:28).

I am secure and comforted in accepting the love of Christ. "Who shall separate us from the love of Christ? Shall trouble or hardship or persecution or famine or nakedness or danger or sword? . . . No, in all these things we are more than conquerors through him who loved us. For I am convinced that neither

death . . .
    life . . .
        angels . . .
            demons . . .
                present . . .
                    future . . .
                        powers . . .
                           height . . .
                             depth,
                                nor anything else in
all creation, will be able to separate us from the love of God
that is in Christ Jesus our Lord" (Rom. 8:35-39).

Homesick For Heaven!

When our Missy was away at college the first semester, she was
so homesick that the daily calls shot our phone bills sky-high. By the
time Thanksgiving arrived our family couldn't wait to be all together
again.

Homesickness hurts. As Missy's mom, I felt it . . . badly. You
know the kind of pain . . . that way-down-deep kind. It was the kind
that makes me want to just sit and moan. It's similar to an impending
"all-day morning sickness nausea" weary feeling! You can't really ex-
plain what's wrong, you just know something is not right.

A week before Missy's holiday break that first fall, something happened to all of our family. Our spirits rose daily. I ceased my "groaning" because I knew that soon we would all spend the next few days with the ones we love the most in this world.

Missy's phone conversations turned from despair to effervescence and encouragment. "I can make it now," she'd exclaim, "I'm coming home soon!" When I saw that little beige car turn into the driveway of our modest house on the corner lot, I dropped whatever I was doing. I hugged that girl long and hard. Both of us were no longer homesick.

You and I can "make it" even when life doesn't run smoothly. We, too, have the hope of going home soon!

Sometimes God deliberately builds hassles and heartache into each of our lives to help us keep our eyes on our eternal home rather than on our earthly one. He is preparing a place for His redeemed more glorious than we can ever imagine.

The Best Home Show Ever

Human imagination can not comprehend the beauty of the believer's eternal paradise. It would be impossible to imagine the splendor we will behold when we first arrive on location. We do know that heaven is a huge and colorful place, but that is not as important, in the final analysis, as the fact that we will live forever there with God.

The Bible does not tell us every detail of our eternal home. What

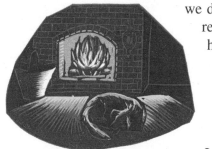

we do know is that everyone who has received Christ as personal Savior has become a child of God (John 1:12) and now possesses eternal life in heaven (John 5:24). The central focus of heaven will not be the walls, streets, or gates, but rather the Lamb of God and His throne. John noted a beautiful emerald green rainbow surrounding the throne (Rev. 4:3). In verse 6 he cited, "Before the throne there was what looked like a sea of glass, clear as crystal."

Heaven will be spotlessly clean and built of transparent gold. The city itself is surrounded by a wall of jasper, as beautiful as a crystal clear diamond, and as brilliant as a transparent icicle in bright sunshine (Rev. 21:18).

With its main street paved with pure gold, heaven's walls rest on 12 foundations inlaid with various precious stones (Rev. 21:21). You and I have toured some magnificent homes before; I've been honored to stay in some bed and breakfast homes that were breathtaking upon arrival. But, oh, dear friend, heaven's colorful elements form a beauty never known to our human eye. Even the finest home shows have not come close to the grandeur we will behold!

What Heaven Is:

Heaven is indescribable: "However, as it is written: No eye has seen, no ear has heard, no mind has conceived what God has prepared for those who love him" (1 Cor. 2:9).

Heaven is incredible: "He will wipe every tear from their eyes. There will be no more death or mourning or crying or pain, for the old order of things has passed away" (Rev. 21:4).

Heaven is instantaneous: "After that, we who are still alive and are left will be caught up together with them in the clouds to meet the Lord in the air. And so we will be with the Lord forever" (1 Thess. 4:17).

Heaven is ingenious: "Now we know that if the earthly tent we live in is destroyed, we have a building from God, an eternal house in heaven, not built by human hands" (2 Cor. 5:1).

Heaven is individual: "Jesus said to her, 'I am the resurrection and the life. He who believes in me will live, even though he dies; and whoever lives and believes in me will never die. Do you believe this?' " (John 11:25-26).

Heaven is indubitable: "Do not let your hearts be troubled. Trust in God; trust also in me. In my Father's house are many rooms; if it were not so, I would have told you. I am going there to prepare a place for you. And if I go and prepare a place for you, I will come back and take you to be with me that you also may be where I am" (John 14:1-3).

What Heaven Is Not:

Heaven has no tears. There will be no more sadness! I don't know about you, but that promise is a thrill to my heart. To instantaneously be at continual peace with no cause for sadness is a blessed thought (Rev. 21:4).

Heaven does not have day and night sequences. Being eternal, time will not be measured by the 24-hour time periods that we know on this earth. Eternity is timeless. Forever literally means "forever." The word itself boggles the human mind. There will be no time barriers nor need for the sun or the moon since there is no day and night (Rev. 21:23-25).

Heaven will not have churches. The

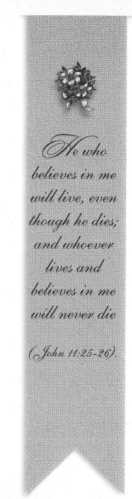

He who believes in me will live, even though he dies; and whoever lives and believes in me will never die

(John 11:25-26).

Bible tells us that the temple was a symbol of the presence of God. Since God himself is present in heaven, there is no need of a temple there (Revelation 21:3). The ultimate community of international believers from every nation and race will worship God together forever in perfect harmony (Rev. 19:1).

Heaven does not have drudgery. We will serve and work in heaven, but the agony and dread of labor will be gone (Rev. 14:13, 22:3). One of the results of sin was the curse of toil and working. In heaven we will enjoy our work. The curse will be gone.

Heaven has no death. Since death means sadness and separation, there is no death in heaven. We will live forever with God and others who die in Christ (Rev. 20:14; 22:3). Sin will be no more; thus death, sin's result, will also be gone forever.

Homeless No More

What awesome truths! Heaven is the wonderful, eternal home of every believer. Unending joy awaits us; separated from earth's impurities and imperfections. Heaven is a place of worship, praise, and service rendered unto our Lord . . . FOREVER!!!

One of the most poignant truths in life is that we all start out homeless. Perhaps I never really understood that statement until I met Lori Ann, a young woman in her late teens. She lived at the shelter for single moms where our Mindy worked last year.

Oh sure, I had seen people on the highway with signs that read, "Help the homeless." Unmoved by their sad faces and silent pleas, I've always driven swiftly by. *Then* I had a name put to one of those faces. When Mindy introduced me to Lori Ann and her precious little baby, Kimberly, that all changed.

Lori Ann made a commitment to Christ and discovered the purpose and joy that He brings. She made room in her life for church, Bible study, and countless opportunities for increasing in knowledge of God and His Word.

I will never forget the night I drove her back to the shelter after a meeting. Instead of complaining about where she was to pillow her head that night, Lori Ann's focus was on the truths she had begun to discover. "I'm no longer homeless!" was her exclamation.

Rather than focusing on the status quo or what she *did not have,* Lori Ann delighted in *what she*

No matter what state your home is in right now, Jesus holds you close to His heart.

knew she did have. Here was a girl who had very little of what this world has to offer. What made a permanent difference in her life each and every day was her new-found hope in Christ. She would never be homeless again — her home awaits her in heaven!

God's love for His people is not determined by the circumstances of our lives. His love is steadfast. Our marital status, career, finances . . . all might fluctuate or break apart. In spite of that, however, we can give thanks for His love toward us. It makes a tremendous difference in how we all approach life.

One of the mansions being prepared in heaven now bears Lori Ann's name and eternal address. Someday, Jesus will welcome her home. He will be her personal guide through each spacious room. No more pressures. No fear of personal failure. No energy, water, financial, or personal crisis there. No wonder she can hardly wait! Me, too! I'm looking forward to that glorious day!

Welcome Home, My Child!

Jesus hasn't forgotten about you! No matter what state your home is in right now, He holds you close to His heart. At this writing, the entire family room in our house is in total disarray due to water leakage. Our electricity went off for hours stopping our sump pump. Groan. Just five minutes ago I groped my way amid the maze of furniture — all shoved to the room's middle allowing carpet along the walls to dry out.

I made my way through the twists and turns and narrow places; thinking of a zillion trails I would have rather trekked along today. It's a pilgrimage I've encountered "far too many times in nine years living in this house," I heard myself grumbling aloud. "Why couldn't we have moved someplace where this didn't happen? Somewhere we didn't have to spend our free time repairing, re-arranging, mopping."

You and I encounter differing struggles. We all take different roads home, each facing our own variety of twists and turns in the road. Do you despair, as I often do, in the journey? Remember, just like God said He would be, He's in control.

He is always up to something in each of our lives. We need only to wait and watch His plan unfold. He is even now preparing a new, wonderful home for each of us, His children. "Do not let your hearts be troubled . . . in my Father's house are many rooms. . . . I am going there to prepare a place for you" (John 14).

Soon, very soon perhaps, the trumpet *will* sound. The Lord himself will descend from heaven with a shout. The dead in Christ will rise first; then we who are alive shall be caught up with them in the clouds to meet the Lord in the air. And so shall we ever be with the Lord!

There is no greater comfort to come home to . . . than knowing our final destination is a glorious home, where we will live forever with the great Comforter!

No sagging body, no cellulite, no weariness nor impending stress. This earthly body will be traded for a brand new, healthy one. Wars, bombings of public buildings, and shootings in schools will be things of the past. We will rest happily in eternal glory cradled in the arms of Jesus' sweet embrace.

Even if the cement is not yet dry on the first brick of your earthly house, don't look down. Look up toward the real estate you hold on high. With open arms, we will be welcomed to a place of comfort beyond the reaches of our imagination. He doesn't care what we look like, where we've been, or who we are. God just cares that we come. He will provide the home and all the comfort our hearts could ever desire.

I can't wait!

You Get by Giving

Have you ever wanted to pass along some hope to a friend, but are still wondering where to go to get a dose for yourself first? A few years ago I learned a secret that has brought a lot of hope, comfort, and joy. Give away the very thing you need the most. Sounds like a paradox, doesn't it? But, it's surprisingly the only sure road to real hope-filled living.

When you are low on funds, give some money (even a small amount) to someone who needs it more. If your four children under six are preventing you from having time alone, then try offering another young mother an afternoon or two a week to care for her children. You'll be thrilled when she reciprocates. Voila! There's your afternoon for time to yourself!

While you're searching for some hope for yourself, become a hope-giver to someone else. We are not to give to get, but it simply works that way following the principle of sowing and reaping. I find that when I give away *something that is precious to me*, to *someone who is precious to me,* I end up receiving much more than I have given!

You can start with something as simple as a note or letter of hope to a friend, "I don't know how you feel, I can't really put myself in your situation,

We will rest happily in eternal glory cradled in the arms of Jesus' sweet embrace.

but I do know what makes me feel better. . . ." Then proceed to tell a story of a time when you felt hopeless and how you got through it. Guess who will be blessed? By giving a gift of hope, you will be blessed as much as your friend!

Look for the hope all around you. It's there! If you are willing to *look,* you will find bright spots in even the darkest day. *But, you have to LOOK!* Hope is everywhere! And you can't out-give God!

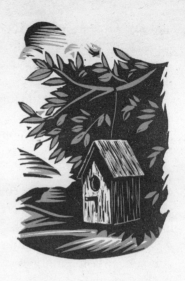

Go looking for hope today. It may be your only chance — you have to *at least try!*

All That Glitters Is Not "Hope"

One day not so long ago, when I was having to *look hard* to find hope, a note came across my desk that made me smile. Along with the smile came laughter and hope. Just when I thought I was the only one in the world who had done irreversible, stupid things, I realized I am not alone. Other women do crazy things, too. Read on. I hope the same smile that came to my face reaches you.

In Melbourne, one of the radio stations paid money ($100-500) for people to tell their most embarrassing stories. This one netted the $500. The winner wrote:

I was due later that week for an appointment with the gynecologist when early one morning I received a call from his office that I had been rescheduled for that morning at 9:30 a.m. I had only just packed everyone off to work and school and it was around 8:45 a.m.

The trip to his office usually took about 35 minutes so I didn't have any time to spare. As most women do, I'm sure, I like to take a little extra effort over hygiene when making such visits, but this time I wasn't going to be able to make the full effort.

So I rushed upstairs, threw off my dressing gown, wet the washcloth and gave myself a wash in "that area" in front of the sink, taking extra care to make sure that I was presentable. I threw the washcloth in the clothes basket, donned some clothes, hopped in the car and raced to my appointment.

I was in the waiting room only a few minutes when he called me in. Knowing the procedure, as I am sure you all do, I hopped up on the table, looked over at the other side of the room and pretended I was in Hawaii or some other place a million miles away from here. I was a little surprised when he said: "My . . . we have taken a little extra effort this morning, haven't we?" But, I didn't respond. With the appointment over, I heaved a sigh of relief and went home.

The rest of the day went normal — some shopping, cleaning, and the evening meal, etc. At 8:30 p.m. that evening my 18-year-old daughter was fixing to go to a school dance, when she called down from the bathroom, "Mom, where's my washcloth?" I called back for her to get another from the cabinet.

She called back, "No, I need the one that was here by the sink, it had all my glitter and sparkles in it."

You see, just about the time you think you're the only one who has ever been humiliated, or hurt, or embarrassed beyond belief . . . think of this *sparkling* woman. What place in your heart do you need to fill with hope today? Fill in the blank: _____. Neither money, possessions, power, education, nor careers can provide the hope you're searching for. Don't waste your time trying to find hope in *things*. Call out to God's love. Nothing else satisfies. When you cry out to Him, "Help," He answers, "I'm already here!"

No one need be hopeless. No one!

Turn Up the Heat

Creating an atmosphere of hope in your home can be likened to regulating your thermostat to set a comfortable temperature inside your house. *Someone* has to punch in the numbers to set a proper degree. Unchecked, you will freeze in the winter and scorch in the summer. Similarly, our homes' emotional climate needs to be properly set. It is then, and only then, that home becomes a restful place where spirits are renewed in a comfortable ambiance.

Just as quickly as the seasons change, so can my home's climate. Left unchecked, our home can go from serene calm to swelling chaos in no time! Just this morning my office began to feel arctic-cold. After putting on socks and a heavy sweater, I finally got smart and turned up the thermostat. Duh! Soon I heard the furnace kicking on to warm things up. Similarly, *I* can become my home's thermostat! When things get ice-cold, instead of giving everyone the cold shoulder, I can turn up the heat! I can be the one who regulates "climate" in my home by setting an atmosphere that renews

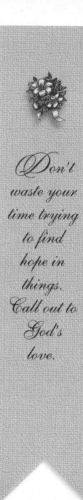

Don't waste your time trying to find hope in things. Call out to God's love.

the spirit physically, spiritually, and emotionally. We all can!

This is especially important on those days when icy winds of hopelessness are blowing strong — frosty gusts. You know those days. You're given the cold shoulder. Emotional icicles hang from the ceiling in every room. Someone needs to turn up the heat. *You* be the one! Infuse your home with HOPE — nothing warms the heart better.

Hope Makes a Difference

HOPE looks for the good in people instead of harping on the worst in them.

HOPE opens doors where despair closes them.

HOPE discovers what can be done instead of grumbling about what cannot be done.

HOPE draws its power from a deep trust in God and the basic goodness of mankind.

HOPE "lights a candle" instead of "cursing the darkness."

HOPE regards problems, small or large, as opportunities.

HOPE cherishes no illusions, nor does it yield to cynicism.

Anonymous

Take Hope — You Are Not Alone!

Nothing can turn a mom to the Lord quite so desperately as seeing her child in pain. I remember standing in the emergency room of a hospital biting the sides of my cheeks until they were shredded as I watched doctors stitching Mindy's bleeding ankle. She was only three years old at the time and *I felt responsible.* Mindy had been riding on the fender of my bicycle and I turned a corner too sharply into loose gravel. I blamed myself for her pain. After all, I *caused* the accident, didn't I?

But that was small compared to the ripping apart of my heart that I experienced years later when Mindy was in trouble and a thousand miles away at college. I found myself stuck in a dark tunnel of despair. Couldn't see even a ray of light at the end. Hopeless. Broken dreams make us feel that way.

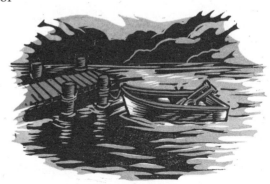

Right now you may be hurting from a broken dream. Hopeless. You haven't even been stitched up yet. In fact, your whole life may seem like an emergency room. Desperately, you want things to change! But, don't know how they can . . . or if they ever will. *It won't last forever!* Whatever you're going through, you can have hope knowing that "this too, shall pass."

You are not facing your future alone.

This poem below by my Mindy says it all so well. She will forever have my inexhaustible thanks to her for surprising me with such a glorious gift at last year's mother-daughter banquet. There was not a dry eye in the auditorium when she finished at the grand piano singing and playing these words to me before four hundred women. May it give you reason to hope, as it has to me and so many.

"I AM NOT ALONE"

Day by day . . .
They've gone so fast
And now I stand here grown.
My world once small
But times have past
And now, I'm on my own.
You've been there with me,

Held my hand tightly.
When I would fall, you'd pick me up.
Then taught me how to stand.
Today I know you differently
Than I've ever known before.
Though you're not always right next to me
I realize more and more
That I am not alone.

When I am weak and *cannot* stand
Now, you can't pick me up.
You've left me to One who can,
That has to be enough.
And when my hand is just too far
You can't hold on — as in the past.
Though it may bring tears
You loosen your loving grasp
And you let me go
Into the arms that can bring me safely home.
There I find you on your knees
And I know . . .
That I am not alone.

Through all my years
You've stood beside me
You walked along life's road.
And then I would often wander
You'd carried my massive load.
But, today my load's too heavy
For even the both of us to bear.
Now, He's waiting to carry me
Because He heard your prayer.
We've created a bond between us
Stronger than the winds that blow.
Though time and miles are against us
This one thing I'll always know —
That I am not alone.
　　　— by Mindy Elaine Hoffman

Instant in Every Season

I was feeling rather smug after having taken advantage of a warm winter day to take down my outdoor holiday decorations. Up and down our block, many of my neighbors had done the same. All but one. I couldn't help noticing the Christmas grapevine wreath still hanging at the top of the garage door of a neighborhood friend's house. Every time I rounded the corner it's message continued to wish passers-by a Merry Christmas. For weeks! *She probably is busy and the Iowa winter now is too rough to be climbing up a ladder,* I thought.

Well into February, with the street covered with snow, I looked up to catch a glimpse of something new attached to the wreath. I practically slid through the icy intersection straining to see what it was that was different about my friend's wreath. It was a bright red heart wishing all "Happy Valentines' Day!"

A few weeks later, the wreath was outlined with green shamrocks throughout March.

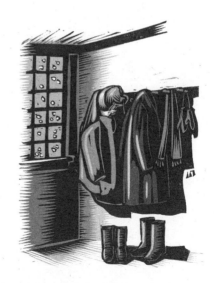

Two weeks before Easter, a pretty yellow ribbon and a darling floppy-eared bunny appeared and stayed throughout April.

The merry month of May came . . . and so did little wooden tulips announcing that spring had finally arrived.

With the warmer weather, I stopped my car one afternoon when I saw Debbie outside her home. I told her how much I'd enjoyed the "changing of the wreath" for the past few months. Even though she and I had not gotten to chat all winter, I told Debbie that I felt as though we had! Her wreath was an almost daily reminder to me of the joy that Debbie is to all she meets. "We have so much to celebrate, I just thought we would celebrate all year long!" she told me.

And celebrate she does! Just being in her presence was a blessing and reminded me that every day, *I can find something to celebrate!* The Lord was using Debbie's wreath as a visual object lesson to minister her life message . . . even when we weren't getting together in person, I was still being blessed by a dear friend who had reason to celebrate all year long.

Similarly, Moses instructed the Israelites to keep annual seasonal celebrations and hang "memorials before their eyes" (Exod. 13:9) so that their families would not forget that the Lord had brought them out of Egypt. They were to celebrate the Passover annually and make certain their children knew why.

Keeping a house is fairly easy; a house is visible. A home is not so visible; thus, keeping a *home* is more difficult. God specifically calls upon women to be the "keepers at home" (Titus 2 :5). One of the ways we can do that is to celebrate what blessings we're enjoying in our lives. Yes, to even hang them on the "doorposts of our homes." May the Lord help us all to hang a wreath on the doorpost of our hearts, reminding even ourselves of the many blessings we have to celebrate.

Believe it or not, by June a red, white, and blue flag appeared and continued on the wreath through July. And in August . . . month after month Debbie's message of cheer rang out!

> Praise the Lord,
>> Praise the Lord,
> Let the earth hear His voice.
>> Praise the Lord,
> Praise the Lord,
>> Let the people rejoice.
> Oh, come to the Father
>> Through Jesus the Son
> And give Him the glory,
>> Great things He hath done!

— Fanny Crosby

And give Him the glory, great things He hath done!

By the Book!

I am no mathematical genius. Believe me, that's putting it mildly. (Take a peek at my checkbook!) When I was in high school, I studied math that was taught during the sixties. After nearly driving numerous teachers to the point of exasperation, I finally made it through algebra and geometry. Much of what I learned is now extinct due to computers and calculators. Unfortunately, the excuse *"I'll never use this!"* never got me out of doing the work while in school. I memorized abhorrent figures, graphs, and measurements that simply no longer exist. Even while assisting my daughters with their homework ten years ago, I was made to see how antiquated my math skills had become.

How thankful I am to know there is one factual equation that makes sense to me. Its validity can never become obsolete because it comes from God's word. The passage is Philippians 4:6-7. No matter how you sum it up, you will arrive at the same answer every time! You won't find it to be a bewildering, rote-memorized mathematic procedure. Even the math-challenged like me can understand this base formula:

$$\textit{Prayer} + \textit{Supplication} + \textit{Thanksgiving} = \textit{PEACE}$$

How well I remember our daughter Missy's frustration when a math assignment consisted not only of the correct answer to a problem, but showing the *proof*, as well. "After all," Mr. Whitehouse would exhort the six-graders, "you don't want to grow up to be a French-fry shoveler all your life!" It was those "proofs" that got to Missy! She would struggle at the kitchen table many a late evening working on draft after draft. And, mind you, Missy was *not exactly her usual perky self* during these intense sessions. "I don't know how I got the answer, *it just works!"* As I recall, the rest of the family was inclined to slip as far away as we all could to escape the frustrating ordeal. By the time her answers began to make sense, Missy would often have filled a wastebasket with wadded papers and endless columns of numerals.

When Missy got stuck on a problem that was beyond both of our reasoning, I'd wearily end my tutorial session with a frustrated "Just go look in the book!" (Promptly I'd then exit the room in delirium.) Now, why didn't we think of that before! It never failed. Later in the evening, Missy would calmly emerge with relief written all over her face and join the family in whatever we were doing.

Sound familiar? Our daily lives are often as complicated as a math problem. Things just don't add up. I'm so glad the formula for peace is not as

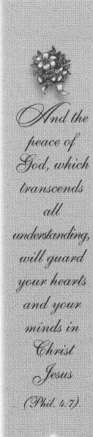

And the peace of God, which transcends all understanding, will guard your hearts and your minds in Christ Jesus

(Phil. 4:7).

difficult, nor does it take so long to find the "proof." That is, IF WE GO TO THE BOOK. We all have doubts, frustrations, and questions that just don't seem to add up . . . no matter how we align the variables. God's peace for us comes to our hearts when we trust in *His* plan for our lives. Not in our own. Life's equation never comes to the right answer when we manipulate the equation to get our own way.

"Be still and know that I am God" (Ps. 46:10) means "Relax, let God figure it out." In times of confusion when we find it difficult to "prove" what's going on — God is still God. He truly knows what is best. His ways are not our ways. I shudder to think how things would have turned out if I had my way in many circumstances of my life. In His loving kindness, God will provide the peace, if we follow the formula.

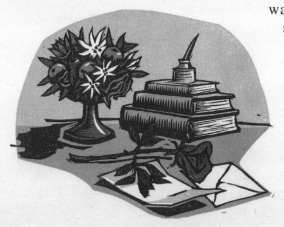

You don't have to know how to add, subtract, multiply, or divide! In Philippians the formula is clear, concise, and constant. It transcends all natural explanations. We may not know *how* it works . . . *"it just works!"* By the Book.

God's Will for Us

Just to be tender, just to be true;
Just to be glad the whole day through.
Just to be merciful, just to be mild;
Just to be trustful as a child.
Just to be gentle and kind and sweet,
Just to be helpful with willing feet.
Just to be cheery when things go wrong,
Just to drive sadness away with a song.
Whether the hour is dark or bright,
Just to be loyal to God and right.
Just to believe that God knows best,
Just in His promise ever to rest;
Just to let love be our daily key,
This is God's will, for you and me.

Anonymous

Some Things Worth Keeping

Rather than having "Aha!" experiences, more often God lets us know His truths in a new and personal way through events in our everyday lives. Such was my reward while attempting to clean the garage last spring. I desired a clean garage, but I didn't want to give up any "stuff." And, girlfriend, we had *lots of stuff!*

Standing at the door measuring from every angle, I realized what Rob had said earlier that morning was right. "No way, no how, are two cars going to fit into our garage next winter unless we get rid of a lot of this stuff!" Rob and I usually feel like we make a pretty good pair. I guess, like a well-fitting pair of shoes, we're a good fit. We walk in stride. But, early in this particular day I knew that I was the one out of step.

Have you ever tried to walk in a pair of high heels when one heel was broken off? Before long, the limping causes you to feel miserable. Rob says that he was attracted to me in college because of my gregarious personality. Little did he know at the time, however, was that sanguines are sentimental pack rats. We want to hold on to everything! Eliminating some of our 26 years of family memories was unthinkable to me! I had tried unsuccessfully for years to part with "treasures" such as the huge stuffed teddy bear that Missy won on the church bus at age five.

As I surveyed the area before attempting the formidable task at hand, I was plagued by a question I've asked myself more than once during the past 26 years. "Why is it that people tend to seek out and marry our opposite?" Sociologists answer that it is universal: We marry someone who has the characteristics we lack. God explains: "the two shall become one flesh" (Gen. 2:24).

In the midst of all my re-arranging, streamlining, sorting, and trashing, God began to reveal one of Rob's great strengths. Acknowledging Rob's sense of order as one of his best inborn traits, I saw where I had allowed it to become a source of contention, rather than blessing. What if we'd both hung on to every sentimental piece of paper or stuffed animal for all these years? No U-Haul truck made would have been able to help haul all the "stuff" out.

And like someone once pointed out: *Even the best things in life are still just things.*

Why then do couples let the very "opposites" that first drew us to one another later become the very sources of painful friction and irritation? With me, I know it's because I want to be right. *My*

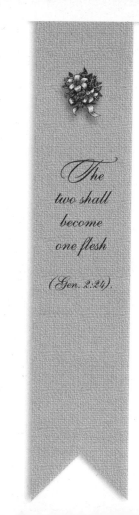

The
two shall
become
one flesh

(Gen. 2:24).

way is best, I say to myself. And there are times when I don't get my way: I let Rob have it with both barrels.

I spent all morning cleaning out the clutter in our garage. I made such a scene, with sorting boxes all up and down our long driveway, a couple of people stopped in their cars to ask if I was having a garage sale. (I probably should have!)

Some items posed a difficult choice — some were tossed; some stayed. More importantly, I chose to clean some attitudes toward Rob that I'd allow to clutter my heart, too. To fulfill an ongoing process of becoming *one,* I needed to take a fresh look at Rob's strengths. I had to admit that our opposites actually add to our joys and togetherness as a couple. It was only a matter of time before I saw the power of that accepting attitude do its work.

It was later that month when Rob and I took a fall foliage trip through eastern Iowa. We had been driving on the highway only a short time when we came within seconds of being part of a serious car accident. Were it not that we were spared by what I believe were God's angels, we would have been hit head-on. Shaken, we stopped by the side of the road to check on those injured and to quiet our nerves.

How thankful I was to have had a fresh reminder in my garage weeks earlier of how special Rob is. I could have lost him without giving him the appreciation he deserves. I simply chose to agree with God that he is an instrument through which God's love becomes evident to me. It's futile when we try to run our homes without God. We run into such big trouble when we do. Try cleaning out some of the "stuff" cluttering your heart today, won't you?

(Added note: Yes, Missy's prized bear made the "cut" . . . one more time!)

Try cleaning out some of the "stuff" cluttering your heart today.

Endnotes

1 Gary Smalley, *Love Languages* (Chicago, IL: Northfield Publishing, 1992).

2 F.J. Wiens, *Her Best for the Master* (Chicago, IL: Moody Press).

About Our Cover Artist

Kit Hevron Mahoney has over 20 years experience as an artist and design professional. She was educated at the University of Colorado, Boulder, and at the Colorado Institute of Art in Denver, where she taught drawing and graphic design for 15 years. She was president/owner of Graphic Creations, Ltd., a national greeting card company and is now part owner of Abend Gallery Fine Art in Denver, where she shows her fine art. Since 1984, her watercolor and pastel landscape and floral paintings have been marketed through a variety of galleries and by private commission. Samples of her work can be viewed at http://home.earthlink.net/~kitm.